Blood Sugar Diet Solution

Joel Oliver

Copyright © 2024 Joel Oliver

Disclaimer:

The information in this book is intended for educational and informational purposes only. The author and publisher make no representations or warranties with respect to the accuracy, applicability, or completeness of the content. The information is provided with the understanding that the author and publisher are not rendering medical, legal, or professional advice. Always seek the advice of a qualified professional with any questions you may have regarding a medical condition or any other subject matter.

Table of Contents

Introduction

Understanding Blood Sugar and Its Importance

Blood sugar (glucose) is an essential source of energy for the body's cells, tissues, and organs. It is the essential fuel that drives all bodily operations, from simple movements to complicated cognitive processes. When we eat carbohydrates, such bread, pasta, fruits, and vegetables, our bodies convert them into glucose, which enters the bloodstream. This process is strictly regulated by insulin, a pancreatic hormone that aids in the transport of glucose from the bloodstream into cells for use or storage.

Maintaining stable blood sugar levels is critical to general health. Fluctuations can cause a variety of health problems, including exhaustion, irritability, difficulty concentrating, and long-term repercussions such as diabetes, cardiovascular disease, and obesity. Chronic high blood sugar, also known as hyperglycemia, can lead to dangerous illnesses including Type 2 diabetes, which occurs when the body becomes resistant to insulin or fails to produce enough insulin. Low blood sugar, often known as hypoglycemia, can induce weakness, confusion, and even loss of consciousness if not treated swiftly.

Understanding blood sugar fluctuations and the factors that influence them—such as nutrition, physical exercise, stress, and sleep—is critical for long-term health. Individuals who learn to manage blood sugar effectively can improve their overall health, lower their risk of chronic diseases, and increase their quality of life.

Overview of the Blood Sugar Diet Solution

The Blood Sugar Diet Solution is a complete method that aims to help people manage their blood sugar levels through food changes, lifestyle changes, and informed decisions. This diet emphasizes whole, nutrient-dense meals while avoiding processed foods and refined sweets, which can cause blood glucose increases. By emphasizing meals that give consistent energy and promote metabolic health, this diet attempts to develop long-term health and wellness.

This solution includes an organized meal plan, recipes, and practical advice for making nutritional adjustments. It promotes the consumption of high-fiber meals, healthy fats, and lean proteins, which help to enhance insulin sensitivity and blood sugar control. In addition, the diet encourages regular physical activity and stress management approaches to improve overall metabolic health.

The Blood Sugar Diet Solution is more than simply a meal plan; it is a lifestyle change that allows people to take control of their health. This program builds the groundwork for better living by educating participants on how food affects blood sugar levels and providing them with the tools they need to make educated decisions.

Who Can Benefit from This Diet?

The Blood Sugar Diet Solution is useful for a wide spectrum of people, especially those who:

1. **Are At Risk for Diabetes**: Those with prediabetes or a family history of Type 2 diabetes can benefit greatly from following this diet. Individuals who make dietary changes early in life can help avoid the onset of diabetes and enhance their overall health.
2. **Struggle with Blood Sugar Management**: For those with diabetes or other metabolic diseases, this diet can help normalize blood sugar levels. It offers practical meal planning and food selection recommendations to help them manage their condition more effectively.
3. **Experience Energy Fluctuations**: Those who frequently experience weariness, mood swings, or difficulties concentrating may benefit from a blood sugar-stabilizing diet. By avoiding blood sugar spikes and falls, they can maintain consistent energy throughout the day.

4. **Seek Weight Management**: The Blood Sugar Diet Solution focuses on nutritious foods and balanced meals to help individuals lose or maintain a healthy weight. This technique can result in long-term weight loss while increasing overall health.

5. **Desire Improved Overall Health**: Anyone looking to improve their health and well-being can benefit from the concepts mentioned in this diet. Focusing on nutrient-dense foods, physical activity, and mindful eating leads to a healthy lifestyle that promotes long-term vitality.

In conclusion, the Blood Sugar Diet Solution is a comprehensive program designed to satisfy the demands of a variety of people, making it an invaluable resource for anyone wishing to improve their blood sugar management, improve their health, and live a more balanced lifestyle. Whether you are at risk for diabetes, are managing a diagnosis, or simply want to improve your health, this diet can provide the information and support you need to succeed.

Chapter 1

The Science of Blood Sugar

What is Blood Sugar?

Blood sugar, often known as blood glucose, is the concentration of glucose in the bloodstream. Glucose is a simple sugar that provides energy for the body's cells. It is largely derived from the carbs we eat, such as fruits, grains, vegetables, and milk. Carbohydrates are digested and converted into glucose, which enters the bloodstream and raises blood sugar levels.

The body relies on a precise glucose balance to function properly. Blood sugar levels fluctuate during the day due to a variety of factors such as dietary intake, physical activity, and hormonal changes. Normal fasting blood sugar levels are normally between 70 and 99 mg/dL. Levels beyond this range may suggest prediabetes or diabetes, while levels below indicate hypoglycemia.

Understanding blood sugar is critical for sustaining energy, cognitive function, and overall wellness. When blood sugar is too high or too low, it can cause a variety of symptoms and long-term health problems.

The Role of Insulin

Insulin is a hormone generated by the pancreas that helps regulate blood sugar levels. After eating, blood sugar levels rise, causing the pancreas to produce insulin into the bloodstream. Insulin increases glucose uptake into cells, where it is utilized for energy or stored for later use. This procedure aids in lowering blood sugar levels back to normal.

Insulin also helps the liver store extra glucose as glycogen, which may then be turned back into glucose when the body needs more energy. In addition, insulin limits the liver's manufacture of glucose, which helps to regulate blood sugar levels.

Insulin resistance occurs when the cells in the body become less responsive to insulin, resulting in high blood sugar levels. Over time, the pancreas may struggle to produce enough insulin to meet the body's needs, culminating in Type II diabetes. Understanding how insulin works is critical for controlling blood sugar levels and avoiding diabetes complications.

Factors Affecting Blood Sugar Levels

Several factors influence blood sugar levels, and understanding them can help people make better dietary and lifestyle decisions. Key elements include:

1. **Diet**: Food choices and quantity have a direct impact on blood sugar levels. Carbohydrate-rich diets, particularly refined sugars and processed foods, can produce fast increases in blood glucose levels. In contrast, high-fiber diets, whole grains, and healthy fats help to maintain stable blood sugar levels.
2. **Physical Activity**: Regular exercise improves insulin sensitivity and glucose utilization. Physical activity can also assist reduce blood sugar levels during and after exercise by increasing glucose absorption into muscle cells.
3. **Stress**: Stress causes the release of chemicals including cortisol and adrenaline, which can raise blood sugar levels. Chronic stress can lead to insulin resistance and impair blood sugar control.

4. **Sleep**: Poor or insufficient sleep might alter blood sugar regulation. Lack of sleep can promote insulin resistance, making it more difficult for the body to control glucose levels adequately.

5. **Medications**: Certain medications, such as corticosteroids and psychiatric treatments, may impact blood sugar levels. Individuals using these drugs should check their blood sugar levels and cooperate with their healthcare professionals to control any variations.

6. **Hormonal Changes**: Menstrual cycles, pregnancy, and menopause might impact insulin sensitivity and blood sugar levels.

Understanding these characteristics can help people make lifestyle adjustments that promote better blood sugar management and general health.

How Blood Sugar Impacts Overall Health

Maintaining stable blood sugar levels is critical to general health and well-being. Chronic high blood sugar, or hyperglycemia, can cause a variety of health concerns, including:

1. **Diabetes**: Persistent high blood sugar levels can lead to Type 2 diabetes, which is characterized by insulin resistance and inadequate production. This syndrome raises the possibility of problems like cardiovascular disease, kidney damage, and nerve damage.

2. **Weight Gain**: Uncontrolled blood sugar levels can lead to weight growth and obesity, specifically abdominal fat. Excess body weight exacerbates insulin resistance, resulting in a tough cycle to reverse.

3. **Cardiovascular Health**: High blood sugar levels can harm blood vessels, increasing the risk of cardiovascular disorders like heart attacks and strokes. Elevated blood sugar can also lead to high blood pressure and high cholesterol levels.

4. **Cognitive Function**: Changing blood sugar levels can impact brain health and function. According to research, diabetics may be more likely to acquire cognitive decline and illnesses such as Alzheimer's disease.

5. **Mood and Mental Health**: Blood sugar abnormalities affect mood and mental health. Low blood sugar levels can cause irritation, anxiety, and weariness, whilst high levels can make you feel sluggish and lethargic.

6. **Inflammation**: High blood sugar levels can cause inflammation in the body, leading to chronic disorders like autoimmune and metabolic syndrome.

To summarize, understanding the science of blood sugar—its definition, insulin's role, the factors that influence it, and the overall health implications—is critical for everyone looking to enhance their health and well-being. Individuals who take proactive actions to maintain blood sugar levels can improve their quality of life and lower their risk of chronic diseases.

Chapter 2

Identifying Blood Sugar Issues

Symptoms of Blood Sugar Imbalance

Recognizing the symptoms of blood sugar imbalance is critical for timely diagnosis and successful management. Blood sugar levels that are very high (hyperglycemia) or low (hypoglycemia) can cause a variety of physical and psychological problems. Common symptoms include:

1. **Hyperglycemia (High Blood Sugar)**:
   - **Increased Thirst:** High blood sugar levels can cause dehydration and dry mouth.
   - **Frequent Urination:** The kidneys remove excess glucose through urine, leading to excessive urination.
   - **Fatigue:** Chronic fatigue can result from cells' inability to access glucose for energy.
   - **Blurred Vision:** High blood sugar levels can cause fluid to drain from the eye lenses, leading to blurred vision and impaired focus.
   - **Headaches:** Fluctuating blood sugar levels may cause headaches and migraines.
   - **Slow Healing:** High glucose levels can impede the body's normal healing process, resulting in delayed recovery from injuries and infections.

2. **Hypoglycemia (Low Blood Sugar)**:

    o **Shakiness**: Trembling and shakiness may occur due to a sudden reduction in blood sugar levels.

    o **Sweating**: Even in cool situations, excessive sweating might occur.

    o **Dizziness or Lightheadedness**: Insufficient glucose may cause dizziness or lightheadedness.

    o **Confusion or Difficulty Concentrating**: Low blood sugar levels can impair cognitive performance, causing disorientation, difficulty focusing, and irritation.

    o **Increased Hunger**: Rapid drops in blood sugar might cause strong hunger and desires for sweet foods.

    o **Mood Changes**: Fluctuating blood sugar levels can cause mood swings, anxiety, and irritation.

Individuals must understand these symptoms in order to proactively check their health. If any of these symptoms recur regularly, it is best to visit a healthcare professional for an evaluation and advice.

Risk Factors for Blood Sugar Disorders

Certain risk factors enhance the possibility of acquiring blood sugar abnormalities, such as Type 2 diabetes and other similar illnesses. Key risk factors are:

1. **Genetics**: A family history of diabetes or blood sugar issues greatly increases the risk. People who have relatives with diabetes are more likely to develop the disease themselves.

2. **Obesity**: Carrying too much weight around the midsection increases the risk of insulin resistance and Type 2 diabetes. Fat tissue can produce hormones that impair insulin's efficacy.

3. **Sedentary Lifestyle**: Lack of physical activity leads to weight gain and insulin resistance. Regular exercise helps to control blood sugar levels by increasing insulin sensitivity.

4. **Poor Diet**: Consuming refined sugars, processed foods, and harmful fats can cause blood sugar rises. A lack of whole foods, fruits, and vegetables can also cause nutrient deficiencies.

5. **Age**: Blood sugar issues are more likely to develop after age 45. Aging might result in decreased physical activity and altered body composition.

6. **Hormonal Changes**: Conditions including PCOS, pregnancy, and menopause can impact insulin sensitivity and blood sugar levels.

7. **Chronic Stress**: Chronic stress can enhance cortisol levels, leading to high blood sugar and insulin resistance.

8. **Sleep Disorders**: Sleep apnea disrupts sleep patterns and consequently affects blood sugar regulation.

By identifying and treating these risk factors, people can take proactive efforts to lower their chances of having blood sugar issues and improve their overall health.

How to Monitor Blood Sugar Levels

Monitoring blood sugar levels is critical for treating blood sugar problems and staying healthy. There are several approaches for properly tracking blood glucose levels:

1. **Self-Monitoring**: Diabetics and others at risk can use a glucometer to monitor their blood sugar levels at home. This entails pricking a fingertip to get a drop of blood and applying it to a test strip that the glucometer reads. Regular monitoring allows people to learn how their diet, physical activity, and medications affect their blood sugar levels.

2. **Continuous Glucose Monitoring (CGM)**: CGM involves inserting a tiny sensor beneath the skin to continually detect glucose levels during the day and night. These gadgets provide real-time data and trends, allowing users to make more educated choices regarding diet and activity.

3. **Lab Tests**: Healthcare practitioners may use laboratory testing to monitor blood sugar levels. Common tests include:
   - **Fasting Blood Sugar Test**: The Fasting Blood Sugar Test measures blood glucose levels after at least 8 hours of fasting. A reading that exceeds 126 mg/dL may suggest diabetes.
   - **Hemoglobin A1c Test**: The Hemoglobin A1c Test assesses average blood sugar levels during the previous 2-3 months. An A1c of 6.5% or higher indicates diabetes.

- o **Oral Glucose Tolerance Test (OGTT)**: The Oral Glucose Tolerance Test (OGTT) monitors blood sugar levels before and after drinking a sweet drink to assess glucose metabolism.

4. **Tracking Symptoms**: Monitor symptoms of high or low blood sugar levels. Keeping a food diary, tracking physical activity, stress levels, and any symptoms you feel will help you manage your blood sugar.

Regular monitoring enables individuals to recognize patterns, make required dietary and lifestyle changes, and work with healthcare specialists to improve blood sugar control.

Understanding Glycemic Index and Load

The glycemic index (GI) and glycemic load (GL) are two key concepts that assist people understand how different foods affect their blood sugar levels.

1. **Glycemic Index (GI)**: The glycemic index ranks carbohydrate-containing foods according to their influence on blood sugar levels. Foods are graded on a scale of 0 to 100, with higher scores suggesting a stronger effect on blood sugar. For example:
   - o **High GI Foods (70 or above)**: High GI meals (70 or above) such as white bread, sugary cereals, and sweets can produce fast rises in blood glucose levels.
   - o **Medium GI Foods (56-69)**: Foods with a medium glycemic index (56-69) include whole grain bread and brown rice.
   - o **Low GI Foods (55 or below)**: Low GI foods (55 or below) such fruits, vegetables, legumes, and whole grains cause a gradual increase in blood sugar levels.

Choosing low to medium GI meals can help maintain stable blood sugar levels, making them a better option for people with blood sugar concerns.

2. **Glycemic Load (GL)**: Considers both a food's GI and the amount of carbohydrates in a normal serving. It gives a more realistic picture of how a particular food would effect blood sugar. To calculate GL, use the formula:

GL=(GI×Carbohydrate content (g))÷100 \text{GL} = \left(\text{GI} \times \text{Carbohydrate content (g)}\right) \div 100GL = (GI × Carbohydrate content (g)) ÷ 100.

- o **Low GL (10 or below)**: Low glycemic load (10 or lower) foods reduce the risk of blood sugar rises.
- o **Medium GL (11-19)**: Foods in the Medium GL range (11-19) have a modest effect on blood sugar levels.
- o **High GL (20 or above)**: Foods with a high glycemic load (20 or higher) should be ingested with caution due to the potential for fast blood sugar rises.

Understanding the glycemic index and glycemic load of foods can help people make healthier choices that promote better blood sugar management. Individuals who focus on low GI and low GL diets can achieve more stable blood sugar levels, minimize cravings, and improve general health.

To summarize, recognizing the signs of blood sugar imbalances, identifying risk factors, learning to successfully monitor blood sugar levels, and knowing the glycemic index and load are all critical stages for people who want to manage their blood sugar and maintain long-term health.

Chapter 3

Nutrition Fundamentals for Blood Sugar Control

Macronutrients: Carbohydrates, Proteins, and Fats

Understanding macronutrients is critical for managing blood sugar levels effectively. Each macronutrient has a distinct role in the body and affects blood sugar management differently.

1. **Carbohydrates**:
   - **Role**: Carbohydrates are the body's main source of energy. When ingested, they convert to glucose, which enters the bloodstream and boosts blood sugar levels.
   - **Types**: There are two types of carbohydrates: simple and complex.
     - **Simple Carbohydrates**: Sugar-sweetened beverages, sweets, and fruits contain simple carbohydrates, which can produce rapid blood sugar rises.
     - **Complex Carbohydrates**: Complex carbohydrates, found in whole grains, legumes, and vegetables, are absorbed slowly, resulting in steady increases in blood sugar.

- o **Recommendations**: To maintain stable blood sugar levels, consume high-fiber, complex carbohydrates and restrict simple sugars and processed grains.

2. **Proteins**:
   - o **Role**: Proteins have critical roles in tissue healing, enzyme and hormone production, and immunological function. They have minimal effect on blood sugar levels.
   - o **Sources**: Sources include lean meats, poultry, fish, eggs, dairy products, legumes, nuts, and seeds.
   - o **Recommendations**: Incorporating protein with carbohydrate-rich meals can decrease glucose absorption, resulting in more stable blood sugar levels.

3. **Fats**:
   - o **Role**: Fats give concentrated energy and aid in absorbing fat-soluble vitamins (A, D, E, and K). They also play an important function in hormone synthesis and cell membrane structure.
   - o **Types**:
     - **Healthy Fats**: Consume healthy fats like olive oil, avocados, nuts, seeds, and fatty seafood.
     - **Unhealthy Fats**: Processed and fried foods high in trans and saturated fats can harm heart health and insulin sensitivity.
   - o **Recommendations**: Choose healthy fats and limit saturated and trans fats for better health and blood sugar management.

Maintaining optimal blood sugar levels and overall health requires a well-balanced diet rich in carbohydrates, proteins, and fats.

Essential Vitamins and Minerals

Vitamins and minerals play crucial roles in supporting metabolic processes and overall health, particularly for those managing blood sugar levels. Key nutrients include:

1. **Chromium**: This mineral improves insulin sensitivity and aids in carbohydrate metabolism. Chromium-rich foods include whole grains, nuts, and green vegetables.

2. **Magnesium**: Low magnesium levels are linked to insulin resistance. Magnesium-rich foods include leafy greens, nuts, seeds, whole grains, and beans.

3. **Vitamin D**: Adequate vitamin D levels are associated with enhanced insulin sensitivity and overall metabolic health. Fatty fish, fortified dairy products, and sunshine exposure are also potential sources.

4. **B Vitamins** B vitamins, specifically B6, B12, and folate, help with energy metabolism and red blood cell synthesis. Whole grains, legumes, and green vegetables are all great sources.

5. **Zinc**: This mineral is required for insulin production and secretion. Zinc-rich foods include beef, seafood, legumes, seeds, and nuts.

A well-balanced diet rich in these vital vitamins and minerals can help regulate blood sugar levels and promote overall health.

Importance of Fiber in Blood Sugar Management

Fiber is an essential component of a balanced diet, especially for controlling blood sugar levels. There are two kinds of dietary fiber: soluble and insoluble.

1. **Soluble Fiber**:
   - **Role**: Soluble fiber dissolves in water, creating a gel-like substance in the digestive tract. It inhibits digestion and glucose absorption, which helps to maintain blood sugar levels.
   - **Sources**: Sources include oats, legumes, fruits (e.g. apples and citrus), and barley.

2. **Insoluble Fiber**:
   - **Role** Insoluble fiber helps bulk up the stool and promotes regular bowel motions. While it has little direct impact on blood sugar levels, it does help with general digestive health.
   - **Sources**: Sources include whole grains, nuts, seeds, and fruit/vegetable skins.

Benefits of Fiber for Blood Sugar Control:

- **Slows Digestion**: Fiber slows carbohydrate digestion, reducing blood sugar rises after meals.
- **Increases Satiety**: Fiber-rich foods increase satiety, reducing appetite and calorie consumption.
- **Improves Gut Health**: A healthy gut flora promotes metabolic health and insulin sensitivity, essential for blood sugar control.

The American Diabetes Association advises a daily fiber intake of at least 25 grams for women and 38 grams for men. Consuming a variety of fiber-rich foods can improve blood sugar management and overall health.

Meal Timing and Frequency

Meal timing and frequency can have a substantial impact on blood sugar regulation. Understanding how and when to eat can help people better manage their blood sugar levels.

1. **Regular Meal Patterns**:
   - Consistent meal timing can improve blood sugar regulation. Skipping meals or eating inconsistently can cause blood sugar changes, making management more difficult.
   - Aim for three balanced meals per day, plus healthy snacks as needed. This method can help prevent excessive hunger and lower the danger of overeating.
2. **Balanced Meals**:
   - To maintain healthy blood sugar levels, meals should contain a variety of macronutrients such as carbohydrates, proteins, and fats. For example, combining a carbohydrate-rich diet (such as brown rice) with a protein source (such as chicken) and healthy fats (such as avocado) can slow digestion and reduce blood sugar fluctuations.

3. **Pre- and Post-Workout Nutrition**:
    o Regular exercisers should plan their meals around their workouts. Before exercising, eat a balanced breakfast or snack rich in carbohydrates and protein to offer energy and prevent low blood sugar. A post-workout meal replenishes glycogen stores and promotes recuperation.

4. **Intermittent Fasting**:
    o Research indicates that intermittent fasting may enhance insulin sensitivity and manage blood sugar levels. However, this strategy should be handled with caution and in consultation with a healthcare expert, particularly for people with diabetes or other health concerns.

5. **Listening to Hunger Cues**:
    o Paying attention to hunger and satiety signals can help prevent overeating or undereating. Eating consciously, or focusing on the flavor and texture of food, might improve digestion and meal satisfaction.

To summarize, understanding nutrition fundamentals, such as the roles of macronutrients, key vitamins and minerals, fiber, and meal time, is critical for successful blood sugar regulation. Individuals can improve their general health and blood sugar control by making informed dietary choices and developing good eating habits.

Chapter 4

Creating Your Blood Sugar-Friendly Meal Plan

Setting Your Goals: Weight Loss vs. Maintenance

Before developing a blood sugar-friendly meal plan, it is critical to establish clear and achievable goals. These goals can vary depending on the individual's needs, such as weight loss, maintenance, or overall health improvement.

1. **Weight Loss Goals**:
   - **Understanding Caloric Deficit**: Losing weight requires consuming less calories than you burn. A 500-750 calorie deficit per day can result in a safe and lasting weight loss of 1-2 pounds per week.
   - **Nutrient Density**: Choose nutrient-dense foods that give critical vitamins and minerals without excessive calories. Prioritize nutritious foods like veggies, lean proteins, whole grains, and healthy fats.

- o **Monitoring Progress**: Monitor progress by tracking weight loss, energy levels, and blood sugar measurements to evaluate meal plan success. Adjust quantities and dietary choices as needed to meet goals.

2. **Maintenance Goals**:
   - o **Caloric Balance**: After achieving a healthy weight, focus on sustaining it. Calculate your daily caloric demands based on your level of exercise to determine how many calories you should consume.
   - o **Sustaining Healthy Habits**: To maintain healthy habits, prioritize nutrient-dense foods and allow yourself occasional pleasures. Maintaining a balanced diet is critical for long-term success and good health.
   - o **Mindful Eating**: Mindful eating involves paying attention to hunger and satisfaction cues to prevent overeating and promote long-term maintenance.

Individuals can construct a tailored meal plan that addresses their specific needs while also promoting blood sugar management by defining clear targets.

Building Balanced Meals

Creating balanced meals is critical for maintaining stable blood sugar levels and providing the body with important nutrients. A balanced meal often contains a variety of macronutrients (carbohydrates, proteins, and fats), as well as fiber and vital vitamins and minerals. Here's how to create a balanced plate:

1. **Carbohydrates (40-50% of the meal)**:
   - o Choose fiber-rich carbs such whole grains (brown rice, quinoa, whole wheat pasta), legumes (beans, lentils), and starchy vegetables (sweet potatoes, peas).
   - o To prevent blood sugar rises, aim for a carbohydrate serving at each meal and limit portion sizes.
2. **Proteins (20-30% of the meal)**:
   - o Include lean protein sources such skinless chicken, fish, tofu, lentils, and low-fat dairy. Protein helps to regulate blood sugar levels and promotes fullness.
   - o Protein servings should be approximately the size of a deck of cards or your palm.

3. **Healthy Fats (20-30% of the meal)**:
    - Include healthy fats from avocados, nuts, seeds, olive oil, and fatty fish (e.g., salmon, mackerel). Healthy fats boost insulin sensitivity and contribute to cardiovascular health.
    - The recommended serving size for fats is one tablespoon for oils and a small handful for nuts and seeds.
4. **Fiber**:
    - Incorporate colorful vegetables into your meals for fiber, vitamins, and minerals. Non-starchy veggies including leafy greens, bell peppers, broccoli, and carrots are wonderful options.
    - To obtain enough fiber, aim for at least 5 servings of veggies and fruits every day.
5. **Sample Balanced Meal**:
    - **Breakfast:** Breakfast includes scrambled eggs with spinach (protein and vegetables), whole grain toast (carbohydrates), and avocado (healthy fat).
    - **Lunch:** Quinoa salad with chickpeas (carbs + protein), mixed greens and tomatoes (vegetables), drizzled with olive oil (good fats).
    - **Dinner:** Dinner consists of grilled chicken breast (protein), roasted sweet potatoes (carbohydrates), and steamed broccoli (vegetables), topped with almonds for added health benefits.

Individuals can efficiently maintain their blood sugar levels while feeling pleased and energized by ensuring that each meal has a balanced ratio of macronutrients and fiber.

Portion Control Techniques

Portion control is essential for controlling blood sugar levels and meeting weight reduction or maintenance targets. Here are some successful portion control techniques:

1. **Use Smaller Plates and Bowls:** Eating from smaller dishes gives the impression of greater servings, which helps to reduce overeating.

2. **Measure Servings:** At first, measuring portions with a food scale or measuring cups will help you grasp the appropriate serving sizes. Individuals can gradually learn to estimate portion amounts without measuring.

3. **Practice Mindful Eating**: Eat slowly and without distractions. Take time to savor each bite, which can boost satisfaction and aid in recognizing hunger signs.

4. **Fill Half Your Plate with Vegetables:** When making meals, try to fill half of the plate with non-starchy vegetables, which are low in calories but high in volume and nutrients.

5. **Divide Meals into Portions:** When preparing meals, try separating bigger amounts into smaller containers for later meals or snacks. This can help you limit your portion sizes and avoid eating on impulse.

6. **Listen for Hunger Cues:** Pay attention to your body's hunger cues. Eat when you're hungry and stop when you're full, rather than completing everything on your plate.

7. **Plan for Snacks:** Eat healthy snacks in between meals to help you stay energized and avoid hunger. Snack quantities should be kept under control, with a focus on protein and fiber.

Individuals who use these portion control approaches can better regulate their food intake, improve blood sugar control, and achieve their health goals.

Sample Meal Plans for Different Calorie Levels

Creating sample meal plans might help people comprehend how to follow a blood sugar-friendly diet while still fulfilling their caloric requirements. The meal plans listed below are adjusted to different calorie levels: 1,500, 1,800, and 2,200.

1,500 Calorie Meal Plan

- **Breakfast:**
    - Serve 1/2 cup cooked oats with 1/2 banana and 1 tablespoon almond butter.
    - One hard-boiled egg

- **Snack:**
    - One small apple
- **Lunch:**
    - Prepare a mixed green salad with grilled chicken, cherry tomatoes, cucumbers, 1/4

avocado, and 1 tablespoon olive oil/vinegar dressing.
  - One slice of whole grain bread
- **Snack**:
  - 1/4 cup hummus with carrot and celery sticks

- **Dinner**:
  - 4 oz baked salmon
  - 1 cup quinoa
  - 1 cup steamed broccoli
- **Evening Snack**:
  - One small unsweetened Greek yogurt

1,800 Calorie Meal Plan

- **Breakfast**:
  - Two scrambled eggs with spinach and tomatoes.
  - Serve 1 slice whole grain toast with 1 tbsp avocado
- **Snack**:
  - 1 medium pear with 1 tablespoon peanut butter
- **Lunch**:
  - Quinoa bowl with 1/2 cup cooked quinoa, 1/2 cup black beans, salsa, and 1/4 avocado
  - Side of mixed greens with lemon vinaigrette
- **Snack**:
  - 1/2 cup cottage cheese with a handful of berries
- **Dinner**:
  - 5 oz grilled chicken breast
  - 1 medium baked sweet potato
  - 1 cup green beans
- **Evening Snack**:
  - 1 oz dark chocolate (70% cocoa or higher)

2,200 Calorie Meal Plan

- **Breakfast**:
  - Make a smoothie with 1 cup unsweetened almond milk, 1 banana, 1/2 cup spinach, 1 tablespoon chia seeds, and 1 scoop protein powder

- **Snack**:
  - 1 small orange and a handful of walnuts (about 1 oz)
- **Lunch**:
  - Turkey wrap with whole grain tortilla, 3 oz turkey breast, 1 slice cheese, lettuce, tomato, and mustard
  - Side of baby carrots
- **Snack**:
  - 1/4 cup trail mix (nuts and dried fruit)

- **Dinner**:
  - 6 oz grilled shrimp or fish
  - 1 cup brown rice
  - 1 cup mixed steamed vegetables (broccoli, carrots, bell peppers)
- **Evening Snack**:
  - 1/2 cup unsweetened Greek yogurt with 1 tablespoon honey and cinnamon

These sample meal plans offer a foundation for preparing balanced, blood sugar friendly meals that match individual calorie requirements. Adjustments can be made to accommodate personal preferences, dietary limitations, and special health goals.

In conclusion, developing a blood sugar-friendly meal plan entails setting specific goals, preparing balanced meals, exercising portion control, and using sample meal plans as inspiration. Individuals who make intelligent meal choices and incorporate a variety of nutrient-dense foods can effectively manage their blood sugar levels and improve their overall health.

Chapter 5

Foods to Include in Your Diet

Incorporating the correct items into your diet is critical for regulating blood sugar and improving overall health. This chapter discusses the greatest foods for blood sugar regulation, superfoods that promote metabolism, healthy snack options for long-lasting energy, and the value of hydration.

Best Foods for Stabilizing Blood Sugar

Choosing the correct foods has a big impact on blood sugar stability. Here are some of the top options to incorporate into your diet:

1. **Non-Starchy Vegetables**:
   o **Examples**: Leafy greens (spinach, kale), broccoli, bell peppers, cauliflower, zucchini.
   o **Benefits**: Low in calories and carbs, but high in fiber and minerals. They promote satiety and lower overall calorie consumption.
2. **Whole Grains**:
   o **Examples**: Quinoa, brown rice, barley, farro, whole oats.

- o **Benefits**: High fiber content and lower glycemic index compared to processed grains promote slower digestion and stable blood sugar levels.

3. **Legumes**:
    - o **Examples**: Lentils, chickpeas, black beans, kidney beans.
    - o **Benefits**: Legumes provide protein, fiber, and complex carbs, which decrease sugar absorption in the bloodstream.

4. **Lean Proteins**:
    - o **Examples**: Skinless poultry, fish, tofu, tempeh, eggs.
    - o **Benefits**: Proteins boost satiety and stabilize blood sugar levels by slowing digestion.

5. **Healthy Fats**:
    - o **Examples**: Avocados, nuts (almonds, walnuts), seeds (chia, flaxseed), olive oil.
    - o **Benefits**: Healthy fats include improved insulin sensitivity and slower glucose absorption, which helps regulate blood sugar levels.

6. **Berries**:
    - o **Examples**: Blueberries, strawberries, raspberries, blackberries.
    - o **Benefits**: Berries are high in antioxidants, fiber, and low in sugar, making them beneficial for reducing inflammation and improving insulin sensitivity.

7. **Fermented Foods**:
    - o **Examples**: Yogurt, kefir, sauerkraut, kimchi.
    - o **Benefits**: Probiotic-rich diets promote intestinal health, which helps regulate blood sugar levels.

Incorporating a mix of these foods into your regular diet can help keep your blood sugar levels stable and support overall health.

Superfoods to Boost Metabolism

Certain meals are referred to as "superfoods" because of their capacity to boost metabolism and aid in weight management. Here are some important superfoods to consider:

1. **Green Tea**:
   - o **Benefits**: Contains catechins, which can boost fat burning and metabolic rate. Regular consumption may improve overall weight loss attempts.
2. **Chili Peppers**:
   - o **Benefits**: Capsaicin in chili peppers increases metabolism and promotes fat oxidation. Including spicy foods can boost calorie expenditure.
3. **Apple Cider Vinegar**:
   - o **Benefits**: Benefits of Apple Cider Vinegar include improved insulin sensitivity and reduced blood sugar levels following meals. It can also aid with appetite management when taken before meals.
4. **Cinnamon**:
   - o **Benefits**: Improves insulin sensitivity and reduces blood sugar levels. Adding cinnamon to dishes can improve flavor while also providing health advantages.
5. **Leafy Greens**:
   - o **Benefits**: High in fiber and low in calories, leafy greens induce a sensation of fullness, aiding in weight management.
6. **Quinoa**:
   - o **Benefits**: Quinoa is a complete protein with a low glycemic index, providing sustained energy and maintaining steady blood sugar levels.
7. **Fatty Fish**:
   - o **Examples**: Salmon, mackerel, sardines.
   - o **Benefits**: Omega-3 fatty acids can boost metabolic health and reduce inflammation, leading to better blood sugar control.

Incorporating these superfoods into your diet can improve metabolic function, aid in weight management, and regulate blood sugar levels.

Healthy Snacks for Sustained Energy

Snacking can be an effective approach for sustaining energy and avoiding blood sugar spikes throughout the day. Here are some healthy snack alternatives that encourage continuous energy:

1. **Nuts and Seeds**:
   - **Examples**: Almonds, walnuts, chia seeds, pumpkin seeds.
   - **Benefits**: Nuts and seeds contain healthful fats, protein, and fiber, providing sustained energy and stabilizing blood sugar levels.

2. **Greek Yogurt with Berries**:
   - **Benefits**: High in protein and antioxidants, this snack promotes digestive health and regulates blood sugar levels.

3. **Veggies with Hummus**:
   - **Examples**: Carrots, celery, bell peppers.
   - **Benefits**: This combo contains fiber, healthy fats, and protein, making it a nutritious snack.

4. **Apple Slices with Nut Butter**:
   - **Benefits**: A balanced snack with fiber, healthy fats, and protein from nut butter will help sustain energy levels.

5. **Cottage Cheese with Pineapple**:
   - **Benefits**: High protein content - Pineapple fiber adds sweetness without causing blood sugar spikes.

6. **Hard-Boiled Eggs**:
   - **Benefits**: Hard-boiled eggs are a protein-rich snack that helps keep you full between meals.

7. **Smoothies**:
   - **Examples**: Combine spinach, protein powder, and a small amount of fruit.
   - **Benefits**: Smoothies offer a balanced mix of nutrients and can be personalized with fruits, veggies, and healthy fats.

Incorporating these healthy snacks into your regular routine can help you maintain consistent energy levels and achieve your blood sugar management objectives.

Hydration: Importance of Water and Low-Calorie Drinks

Staying hydrated is critical for overall health and has a substantial impact on blood sugar regulation. Here's why hydration is important and some advice for selecting healthy beverage choices:

1. **Importance of Water**:
   - **Blood Sugar Regulation**: Water is important for blood sugar regulation as it helps kidneys wash away extra sugar from the bloodstream. Staying hydrated can help you maintain stable blood sugar levels.
   - **Satiety**: Drinking water before meals can increase satiety and minimize calorie intake.

2. **Low-Calorie Drinks**:
   - **Herbal Teas**: Herbal teas, which are caffeine-free and generally high in antioxidants, can give hydration without the addition of sugar. Chamomile, peppermint, and rooibos are excellent possibilities.
   - **Sparkling Water**: Sparkling water, a delightful alternative to sugary drinks, can be consumed simply or with fresh fruits, herbs, or citrus for extra flavor.
   - **Diluted Fruit Juices**: If you enjoy juice, dilute it with water to lower sugar level and maintain flavor.

3. **Avoiding Sugary Drinks**:
   - **Sodas and Sweetened Beverages**: These high-calorie drinks might induce abrupt blood sugar increases. Choose unsweetened beverages whenever possible.
   - **Alcohol**: Moderate alcohol consumption can contribute to a balanced diet, but it's crucial to limit the type and amount consumed. Choose low-calorie alternatives and avoid sugary mixers.

4. **General Hydration Tips**:
   - Drink at least 8 cups (64 ounces) of water everyday, adjusting for activity level and weather.

- o Carry a reusable water bottle to maintain consistent water intake throughout the day.
- o Monitor urine color: mild yellow suggests enough hydration, while dark yellow may signal a need for additional fluids.

Individuals can improve their general health and regulate their blood sugar more effectively by focusing on hydration with water and low-calorie beverages.

Incorporating the correct items into your diet is an essential step toward controlling blood sugar levels and improving overall health. Individuals can achieve a balanced and effective diet by focusing on nutrient-dense foods, superfoods that improve metabolism, nutritious snacks for prolonged energy, and adequate hydration. Making informed food choices and adopting good eating habits can result in better blood sugar control and a healthier lifestyle.

Chapter 6

Foods to Avoid

Managing blood sugar levels requires both understanding what to eat and identifying what to avoid. This chapter discusses high glycemic index foods, the negative consequences of processed foods, how to find hidden sugars, and how alcohol affects blood sugar levels.

High Glycemic Index Foods

The glycemic index (GI) is a measure of how quickly a food raises blood glucose levels. Foods having a high GI can induce rapid blood sugar increases, which can be harmful, particularly for people with diabetes or blood sugar disorders. Here are some common high-glycemic-index foods to avoid:

1. **White Bread and Pastries**:
    o **Examples**: Regular white bread, bagels, croissants.
    o **Impact**: Refined flour-based diets can quickly raise blood glucose levels.
2. **Sugary Cereals**:
    o **Examples**: Many breakfast cereals with added sugars.
    o **Impact**: Despite being advertised as healthful, high sugar content in cereals might cause raised blood sugar levels.
3. **White Rice and Pasta**:
    o **Examples**: Regular white rice and pasta prepared with refined flour.

- o **Impact**: Both are easily digested and turned into glucose, causing fast blood sugar increases.

4. **Potatoes**:
   - o **Examples**: Mashed potatoes, French fries, potato chips.
   - o **Impact**: Potatoes have a high glycemic index, leading to considerable blood sugar rises.

5. **Sweets and Candies**:
   - o **Examples**: Gummy candies, chocolates, and sugary snacks.
   - o **Impact**: Sugary, low-nutrient diets can cause blood sugar rises and energy dumps.

6. **Certain Fruits**:
   - o **Examples**: Watermelon, pineapple, and ripe bananas.
   - o **Impact**: Excessive consumption of fruits with a high GI might cause rapid blood sugar spikes, despite their overall health benefits.

Tip: Choose low-GI foods including whole grains, legumes, and most non-starchy vegetables, which release glucose more slowly into the bloodstream

Processed Foods and Their Effects

Processed foods are frequently heavy in harmful fats, carbohydrates, and sodium, and they can have a number of adverse impacts on blood sugar levels:

1. **High in Added Sugars**:
   - o Processed foods including snacks, sauces, and ready-made meals are high in added sugars, which can quickly raise blood sugar levels.

2. **Low Nutritional Value**:
   - o Processed foods generally lack key nutrients, resulting in imbalanced diets and poor health effects. This can make it difficult to maintain consistent blood sugar levels.

3. **Trans Fats and Saturated Fats**:
   - o Processed snacks and fried foods contain trans and saturated fats, which can lead to insulin resistance and impaired blood sugar management.

4. **High Sodium Content**:
   - o High sodium content can cause hypertension and raise the risk of heart disease, especially for diabetics.
5. **Preservatives and Artificial Ingredients**:
   - o Many processed foods contain preservatives and artificial substances that can impact gut health and inflammation, which are linked to blood sugar regulation.

Tip: For improved blood sugar regulation, eat complete, minimally processed foods such fresh fruits and vegetables, whole grains, lean meats, and healthy fats.

Hidden Sugars: Reading Labels Effectively

Understanding food labels is crucial for detecting hidden sugars in processed foods. Here's how to read labels efficiently:

1. **Check the Ingredients List**:
   - o Look for sugars mentioned under various names, such as sucrose, high fructose corn syrup, glucose, fructose, and agave nectar. The closer sugar is to the top of the list, the higher its concentration in the product.
2. **Identify Serving Sizes**:
   - o Refer to the label for serving size information. A product's sugar content may appear low per serving, but if the serving size is small, you may consume more than you anticipate.
3. **Look for Total Sugars**:
   - o The nutrition information panel displays total sugars, which comprise both natural sugars (found in fruits) and added sugars. Look for products with little added sugar.
4. **Watch Out for "Healthy" Labels**:
   - o Products promoted as "low-fat" or "fat-free" may include additional sugars to enhance flavor. Always double-check the ingredient list and nutrition data, regardless of marketing promises.

5. **Beware of Sugar Substitutes**:
   - Even if sugar alternatives are fewer in calories, they might still cause cravings for sweet foods. Be cautious of their impact on your eating habits.

Tip: For improved blood sugar regulation, go for items with few ingredients and no added sugars or artificial sweeteners.

Alcohol and Blood Sugar Levels

Alcohol has complex affects on blood sugar levels, and understanding these effects is critical for anyone managing blood sugar concerns:

1. **Initial Blood Sugar Spike**:
   - Alcoholic beverages with high sugar content, such as sweet wines and cocktails, can induce a fast spike in blood sugar levels.
2. **Subsequent Drop in Blood Sugar**:
   - After the first surge, alcohol consumption can cause a decline in blood sugar levels, particularly when eaten without food. This is because alcohol impairs the liver's capacity to release glucose into the bloodstream.
3. **Risk of Hypoglycemia**:
   - Diabetics on blood sugar-lowering medication, such as insulin or sulfonylureas, may have hypoglycemia (low blood sugar) after consuming alcohol. It is critical to regularly monitor blood sugar levels in this situation.
4. **Caloric Content**:
   - Excessive alcohol consumption might lead to weight gain and complicate blood sugar regulation.
5. **Hydration**:
   - Alcohol can cause dehydration, affecting overall health and complicating blood sugar regulation.

Tip: If you decide to drink alcohol, do it in moderation, choose lower-sugar options, and always pair it with food to help stabilize blood sugar levels.

To maintain stable blood sugar levels, avoid high glycemic index foods, processed foods, hidden sugars, and limit alcohol consumption. Making informed choices about what to eat and what to avoid can have a big impact on your overall health and well-being. Understanding which foods to avoid will help you gain control of your blood sugar levels and support your road to a healthier lifestyle.

Chapter 7

Recipes for Blood Sugar Stability

Maintaining stable blood sugar levels entails not just avoiding specific foods, but also consuming nutritious, tasty meals and snacks. This chapter includes a number of recipes that are specifically designed to promote blood sugar stability. You'll find selections for breakfast, lunch, supper, snacks, and even desserts, all designed to help you enjoy delicious meals while properly managing your blood sugar.

Breakfast Recipes

1. Overnight Chia Seed Pudding

Ingredients:

- 1/4 cup chia seeds
- 1 cup unsweetened almond milk
- 1/2 teaspoon vanilla extract
- Stevia or monk fruit sweetener (to taste)
- Fresh berries for topping

Procedure:

1. In a medium bowl, combine the chia seeds, almond milk, vanilla essence, and sweetener.

2. Stir the mixture thoroughly to ensure that the chia seeds are uniformly distributed.

3. Cover the bowl and refrigerate overnight (or at least 4 hours) until the pudding is thick.

4. In the morning, give the pudding a thorough stir and top with fresh berries before serving.

Time Frame:

- Preparation Time: 5 minutes
- Yield: 1 serving

Nutritional Value (approx.):

- Calories: 180
- Protein: 5g
- Fat: 9g
- Carbohydrates: 20g
- Fiber: 10g

Alternative Ingredients:

- Almond milk can be replaced with coconut milk or soy milk.
- Chia seeds can be replaced with flaxseeds.

2. Vegetable Omelette

Ingredients:

- 2 large eggs or egg whites
- 1/4 cup diced bell peppers
- 1/4 cup chopped spinach
- 1/4 cup diced tomatoes
- Salt and pepper to taste
- Cooking spray or olive oil for the pan

Procedure:

1. In a mixing basin, whisk the eggs or egg whites until fully blended. Season with salt and pepper.

2. Place a nonstick skillet over medium heat and lightly coat with cooking spray or olive oil.

3. Sauté the diced bell peppers for 2-3 minutes, until they are slightly softened.

4. Cook for an additional 1-2 minutes, or until the spinach has wilted.

5. Pour the egg mixture over the sautéed vegetables and heat until the edges set (approximately 2-3 minutes).

6. Carefully flip the omelette and cook for another 1-2 minutes, or until fully set.

7. Transfer the omelette to a platter and serve immediately.

Time Frame:

- Preparation Time: 10 minutes
- Yield: 1 serving

Nutritional Value (approx.):

- Calories: 200
- Protein: 18g
- Fat: 12g
- Carbohydrates: 6g
- Fiber: 2g

Alternative Ingredients:

- Vegan options include egg replacements or silken tofu.
- Customize using your preferred vegetables.

3. Quinoa Breakfast Bowl

Ingredients:

- 1/2 cup cooked quinoa
- 1/4 cup unsweetened Greek yogurt
- 1/4 cup mixed berries (blueberries, raspberries, strawberries)
- 1 tablespoon chopped nuts (almonds, walnuts, or pecans)
- Cinnamon (optional, for flavor)

Procedure:

1. In a mixing dish, combine the cooked quinoa and Greek yogurt until thoroughly blended.
2. Top with mixed berries and chopped nuts.
3. For added taste, sprinkle with a pinch of cinnamon.
4. Serve immediately or refrigerate for an easy breakfast alternative.

Time Frame:

- Preparation Time: 5 minutes
- Yield: 1 serving

Nutritional Value (approx.):

- Calories: 300
- Protein: 14g
- Fat: 10g
- Carbohydrates: 40g
- Fiber: 6g

Alternative Ingredients:

- Quinoa can be replaced with cooked oatmeal or millet.

- Dairy-free yogurt can be used instead of Greek yogurt.

Lunch and Dinner Ideas

4. Lentil and Vegetable Salad

Ingredients:

- 1 cup cooked lentils
- 1 cup diced cucumber
- 1/2 cup cherry tomatoes, halved
- 1/4 cup red onion, diced
- 2 tablespoons olive oil
- 1 tablespoon lemon juice
- Salt and pepper to taste
- Fresh herbs (parsley or cilantro, optional)

Procedure:

1. In a large mixing dish, add cooked lentils, diced cucumber, cherry tomatoes, and red onion.
2. In a separate small bowl, mix together the olive oil, lemon juice, salt, and pepper.
3. Drizzle the dressing over the salad and gently toss to mix.
4. Add chopped herbs if preferred, and serve chilled or at room temperature.

Time Frame:

- Preparation Time: 10 minutes
- Yield: 2 servings

Nutritional Value (approx.):

- Calories: 220
- Protein: 12g
- Fat: 9g
- Carbohydrates: 30g
- Fiber: 12g

Alternative Ingredients:

- Replace lentils with chickpeas or black beans.
- Replace olive oil with avocado oil.

5. Baked Salmon with Asparagus

Ingredients:

- 2 salmon fillets (about 6 oz each)
- 1 bunch asparagus, trimmed
- 2 tablespoons olive oil
- Lemon slices (for garnish)
- Salt and pepper to taste

Procedure:

1. Preheat the oven to 400 °F (200 °C).
2. On a baking sheet, place the salmon fillets and asparagus in a single layer.
3. Season the salmon and asparagus with salt and pepper. Drizzle them with olive oil.
4. Place lemon wedges on top of each salmon fillet.
5. Bake for 12-15 minutes, or until the salmon flaked easily with a fork and the asparagus was soft.
6. Serve hot with lemon slices on the side, if desired.

Time Frame:

- Preparation Time: 5 minutes
- Cooking Time: 15 minutes
- Yield: 2 servings

Nutritional Value (approx.):

- Calories: 350
- Protein: 30g
- Fat: 23g
- Carbohydrates: 8g
- Fiber: 4g

Alternative Ingredients:

- Salmon can be replaced with trout or tilapia.
- Green beans or broccoli can be used instead of asparagus.

6. Zucchini Noodles with Pesto

Ingredients:

- 2 medium zucchinis, spiralized
- 1/4 cup store-bought or homemade pesto
- 1/2 cup cherry tomatoes, halved (optional)
- Grated Parmesan cheese (optional, for topping)

Procedure:

1. In a nonstick skillet, cook the spiralized zucchini noodles over medium heat for 2-3 minutes, or until slightly softened.
2. Remove the skillet from the heat and mix in the pesto until the noodles are thoroughly covered.
3. If using, add the halved cherry tomatoes and gently toss.
4. Serve warm, with optional grated Parmesan cheese.

Time Frame:

- Preparation Time: 10 minutes
- Cooking Time: 5 minutes
- Yield: 2 servings

Nutritional Value (approx.):

- Calories: 150
- Protein: 4g
- Fat: 11g
- Carbohydrates: 10g
- Fiber: 4g

Alternative Ingredients:

- For a different flavor, substitute pesto with marinara sauce.
- Zucchini can be replaced with spaghetti squash.

Snack Recipes

7. Hummus with Vegetable Sticks

Ingredients:

- 1 cup canned chickpeas, drained and rinsed
- 2 tablespoons tahini
- 2 tablespoons olive oil
- Juice of 1 lemon
- 1 garlic clove, minced
- Salt to taste
- Assorted raw vegetables (carrots, celery, bell peppers) for dipping

Procedure:

1. In a food processor, blend the chickpeas, tahini, olive oil, lemon juice, minced garlic, and salt.
2. Blend until smooth, adding a little water as needed to achieve the appropriate consistency.
3. Serve hummus alongside a variety of raw veggies for dipping.

Time Frame:

- Preparation Time: 10 minutes
- Yield: 4 servings

Nutritional Value (approx.):

- Calories: 100 (per serving of hummus)
- Protein: 5g
- Fat: 5g
- Carbohydrates: 10g
- Fiber: 3g

Alternative Ingredients:

- Tahini can be replaced with sunflower seed butter.
- White beans can substitute for chickpeas.

8. Almond Butter Apple Slices

Ingredients:

- 1 apple, sliced
- 2 tablespoons almond butter
- Cinnamon (optional, for flavor)

Procedure:

1. Core the apple and cut it into wedges.
2. Spread almond butter on each apple slice.
3. Sprinkle with cinnamon if desired.
4. Serve immediately as a nutritious snack.

Time Frame:

- Preparation Time: 5 minutes
- Yield: 1 serving

Nutritional Value (approx.):

- Calories: 200
- Protein: 4g
- Fat: 12g

- Carbohydrates: 24g
- Fiber: 4g

Alternative Ingredients:

- Almond butter can be substituted with peanut butter or sunflower seed butter.
- Any type of apple can be used.

9. Greek Yogurt with Nuts and Seeds

Ingredients:

- 1 cup unsweetened Greek yogurt
- 2 tablespoons mixed nuts (almonds, walnuts)
- 1 tablespoon chia seeds or flaxseeds
- Stevia or monk fruit sweetener (to taste)

Procedure:

1. In a bowl, combine Greek yogurt and sweetener to taste.
2. Sprinkle with mixed nuts and chia or flaxseeds.
3. Serve immediately as a nutritious snack.

Time Frame:

- Preparation Time: 5 minutes
- Yield: 1 serving

Nutritional Value (approx.):

- Calories: 250
- Protein: 20g
- Fat: 15g
- Carbohydrates: 10g
- Fiber: 6g

Alternative Ingredients:

- For a dairy-free alternative to Greek yogurt, try coconut yogurt.
- Nuts can be swapped for seeds like pumpkin or sunflower seeds.

Desserts That Won't Spike Your Blood Sugar

10. Cauliflower Rice Stir-Fry

Ingredients:

- 1 small head of cauliflower, grated or processed into rice
- 1 cup mixed vegetables (bell peppers, peas, carrots)
- 2 tablespoons low-sodium soy sauce or tamari
- 1 tablespoon sesame oil
- 1 garlic clove, minced
- Green onions for garnish (optional)

Procedure:

1. Heat the sesame oil in a large skillet over medium heat. Sauté the minced garlic for 30 seconds.
2. Stir in the grated cauliflower and other veggies until thoroughly combined.
3. Cook for 5-7 minutes, until the cauliflower is tender and the veggies are heated thoroughly.
4. Stir in the soy sauce and simmer for an additional minute.
5. Garnish with green onions before serving.

Time Frame:

- Preparation Time: 10 minutes
- Cooking Time: 7 minutes
- Yield: 2 servings

Nutritional Value (approx.):

- Calories: 120
- Protein: 5g
- Fat: 5g
- Carbohydrates: 15g
- Fiber: 5g

Alternative Ingredients:

- Cauliflower rice can be substituted with broccoli rice or brown rice.
- Mixed vegetables can include any preferred choices.

This collection of dishes tries to provide tasty options for breakfast, lunch, supper, snacks, and desserts that can help keep blood sugar levels stable. Each dish emphasizes entire, nutrient-dense ingredients to help you achieve improved blood sugar management without losing flavor or enjoyment. Experiment with these recipes to find your favorites, and then eat a balanced diet to maintain health and vitality.

Chapter 8

Lifestyle Changes for Long-Term Success

Incorporating Physical Activity

Understanding the Role of Exercise Including physical activity in your daily routine is critical for maintaining good blood sugar levels. Regular exercise improves insulin sensitivity, allowing your cells to effectively utilize the glucose in your system. This not only helps with blood sugar control, but also improves overall health, weight management, and mood.

Types of Exercise for Blood Sugar Management

1. **Aerobic Exercise:** Walking, jogging, cycling, and swimming are all examples of aerobic exercise that raises your heart rate and improves cardiovascular health. Aim to complete at least 150 minutes of moderate-intensity aerobic activity every week.

2. **Strength Training:** Strength training increases muscular mass, which can enhance insulin sensitivity. Aim for at least two days of strength training per week, with a focus on main muscle groups.

3. **Flexibility and Balance Exercises:** Activities like yoga and tai chi can help relieve stress while also improving overall balance and flexibility, all of which are good for your long-term health.

Setting Realistic Goals Begin with small, manageable goals, such as going for a 10-minute walk every day and gradually increasing the duration and intensity. Use tools like fitness trackers to track your progress and stay motivated.

Stress Management Techniques

The Impact of Stress on Blood Sugar Chronic stress can cause elevated cortisol levels, which can raise blood sugar levels and encourage poor eating behaviors. Effective stress management practices are essential for maintaining stable blood sugar levels.

Stress Management Strategies

1. **Mindfulness and Meditation:** Practicing mindfulness or meditation can help you relax and reduce stress. Aim for at least 10-15 minutes of mindfulness meditation every day.
2. **Deep Breathing Exercises:** Techniques like diaphragmatic breathing can help reduce tension rapidly. Inhale deeply through your nose, hold for a few seconds before slowly exhaling through your mouth.
3. **Physical Activity:** Regular exercise is a natural stress reducer. It benefits not just physical health, but also emotions and total well-being.
4. **Time Management:** Plan out your daily responsibilities to avoid feeling overwhelmed. Prioritize work and delegate as much as possible to decrease stress.

The Importance of Sleep

Sleep and Blood Sugar Regulation Adequate sleep is essential for good health and is directly related to blood sugar regulation. Poor sleep quality can cause insulin resistance and increased hunger, making it more difficult to maintain normal blood sugar levels.

Tips for Improving Sleep Quality

1. **Establish a Sleep Routine:** Go to bed and wake up at the same time every day to help regulate your body's internal clock.

2. **Create a Relaxing Sleep Environment:** Keep your bedroom dark, cool, and quiet. Consider installing blackout curtains, earplugs, or a white noise machine.

3. **Limit Screen Time Before Bed:** Screens emit blue light, which might interfere with melatonin production. Aim to switch off all screens at least an hour before bedtime.

4. **Watch Your Diet:** Avoid large meals, coffee, and alcohol close to bedtime because these might impair sleep.

Building a Support System

The Role of Support in Lifestyle Changes: A robust support system is essential for long-term success in blood sugar management. Social relationships, whether with family, friends, or support groups, can offer encouragement, accountability, and drive.

Ways to Build Your Support System

1. **Seek Professional Guidance:** Consider consulting with a qualified dietitian or a certified diabetes educator who can offer personalized guidance and assistance.

2. **Join a Support Group:** Connecting with people going through similar experiences can bring useful insights, encouragement, and a sense of belonging.

3. **Involve Family and Friends:** Tell your loved ones about your goals and encourage them to help you in adopting better habits, making the trip more pleasurable and achievable.

4. **Utilize Online Resources:** Many online communities and forums offer support, resources, and advice for efficiently regulating blood sugar levels.

Incorporating these lifestyle changes—regular physical activity, stress management strategies, prioritizing sleep, and developing a supporting network—will greatly improve your long-term blood sugar control. By incorporating these modifications into your everyday routine, you can improve not only your blood sugar control, but also your general quality of life.

Chapter 9

Monitoring and Adjusting Your Plan

How to Track Your Progress

Importance of Monitoring Your Blood Sugar Tracking your progress is an important part of managing your blood sugar effectively. Regularly monitoring your blood sugar levels can provide useful insights into how your nutrition, physical activity, and lifestyle choices affect your health. This information enables you to make informed decisions to improve your blood sugar management strategy.

Methods for Monitoring Blood Sugar

1. **Blood Glucose Meters:** A glucometer allows you to monitor your blood sugar levels at different times of the day. It is critical to test at consistent periods, such as fasting in the morning and after meals.

2. **Continuous Glucose Monitors (CGMs):** CGMs track blood sugar levels in real-time, providing insights into daily changes. They can help you detect patterns and factors that affect your blood sugar.

3. **Journaling:** Keep a food and activity journal to track your diet, exercise, and blood sugar levels. This technique can help you find links between your food, activities, and blood sugar fluctuations.

4. **Apps and Online Tools:** Consider using applications developed to track blood sugar levels and food plans. These tools make data entry and analysis easier by offering graphs and long-term trends.

Setting Baselines and Goals Establish a baseline blood sugar level to determine your starting point. Set achievable short- and long-term goals for improvement. Review your progress on a regular basis and make any necessary adjustments to your goals.

Adjusting Your Diet Based on Results

Understanding Data and Trends As you monitor your blood sugar levels, you may observe patterns that are specific to your food and lifestyle. Analyzing this data will allow you to determine which foods and practices contribute to higher or lower blood sugar levels.

Making Dietary Adjustments

1. **Identify Problem Foods:** If particular foods routinely cause high blood sugar, consider limiting or eliminating them from your diet. Concentrate on learning their glycemic index and how it affects your body.
2. **Experiment with Portion Sizes:** Sometimes the quantity of food has a greater effect on blood sugar than the food itself. Experiment with different portion amounts to achieve the ideal balance for your body.
3. **Incorporate More Low-GI Foods:** To prevent blood sugar spikes, include whole grains, legumes, veggies, and healthy fats in your diet.
4. **Adjust Meal Timing:** Eating smaller, more frequent meals will help stabilize blood sugar levels. Experiment with meal time to see what works best for you.

Evaluating Results After making modifications, continue to monitor your blood sugar levels to see how the changes effect your results. It may take some time to see noticeable benefits, so be patient and wait for incremental changes.

Knowing When to Seek Professional Help

Recognizing the Signs While self-management is necessary, recognizing when to seek expert assistance is as critical. If you encounter any of the following, consider checking with a healthcare provider:

1. **Consistently High or Low Blood Sugar Levels:** If your readings remain outside your target range despite dietary and lifestyle changes, get advice.
2. **Severe Symptoms:** Severe symptoms, including acute exhaustion, frequent urination, increased thirst, or unintended weight loss, require emergency medical intervention.
3. **Difficulty Managing Your Plan:** Seek help from a healthcare expert if you're feeling overwhelmed or unsure about your blood sugar management plan.

Consulting Professionals

1. **Registered Dietitians:** A nutritionist who specializes in diabetes management can assist you in creating a personalized meal plan and providing education on successful blood sugar management.
2. **Endocrinologists:** Endocrinologists offer specialist care and management solutions for diabetes and other blood sugar disorders.
3. **Certified Diabetes Educators:** Certified Diabetes Educators provide assistance on self-management, insulin use (if needed), and blood sugar monitoring.

Monitoring and changing your blood sugar management plan is a continuous process that demands both vigilance and flexibility. By recording your progress, making required adjustments depending on your results, and understanding when to seek professional assistance, you can successfully walk the path to better blood sugar control and general health.

Chapter 10

Success Stories and Tips from the Community

Inspiring Testimonials

Real-Life Transformations Hearing from people who have successfully controlled their blood sugar levels can be really inspiring. Here are a few encouraging testimonials from people who have adopted lifestyle adjustments and found success along the way:

1. **Maria's Journey:** Diagnosed with prediabetes, Maria understood she needed to make significant lifestyle adjustments. She started tracking her meals and adding more healthy foods to her diet. "I started meal prepping and found it much easier to stick to my goals," she told me. Maria shed 25 pounds over the course of a year and drastically improved her blood glucose levels. "I feel more energetic and in control of my health than ever before."

2. **David's Story:** David, a busy professional, struggled to find time for exercise and a balanced diet. After joining a local diabetes support group, he realized the significance of meal scheduling and portion control. "Having a community that understands my challenges has been invaluable," he says. With the help of his group, David introduced short workouts into his daily routine and changed his eating habits. Not only did he control his blood sugar, but he also developed confidence in his capacity to manage his health.

3. **Lisa's Success:** Diagnosed with Type 2 diabetes, Lisa felt overwhelmed by the necessary dietary changes. "I was scared at first, but then I found a nutritionist who helped me create

a realistic meal plan," she claims. Lisa lost 30 pounds and discovered a new love for cooking nutritious meals by focusing on balanced meals and regular exercise. "Now, I see my diagnosis as a chance to improve my life rather than a limitation."

Common Challenges and Solutions

Navigating Obstacles on the Path to Success While each journey is unique, many people confront similar issues when regulating blood sugar. Here are some frequent challenges and practical solutions:

1. **Challenge: Cravings for Sugary Foods**
   - **Solution:** Stock up on nutritious snacks like nuts, seeds, and low-sugar fruits. Also, use natural sweeteners like stevia or monk fruit in moderation to fulfill your sweet appetite without raising your blood sugar.
2. **Challenge: Social Situations and Eating Out**
   - **Solution:** Communicate your dietary preferences to friends and family when eating out. Look through restaurant menus ahead of time to find healthier selections. Consider proposing more nutritional options or organizing a potluck where you can bring a dish.
3. **Challenge: Time Constraints for Meal Prep**
   - **Solution:** Set aside one day per week for meal preparation. Batch prepare grains, meats, and roasted veggies so they may be combined and matched throughout the week. Use slow cookers or Instant Pots for hands-free cooking.
4. **Challenge: Staying Motivated**
   - **Solution:** Set small, attainable goals and praise accomplishments along the way. Connect with others through support groups or online communities where you may share your triumphs and receive encouragement.

Tips from Those Who Have Succeeded

Strategies for Long-Term Success Here are some helpful tips from people who have successfully maintained their blood sugar:

1. **Stay Informed:** Knowledge is power. Continue to educate yourself about blood sugar management, nutrition, and physical activity. Attend workshops, study books, or use reliable internet resources.

2. **Find an Accountability Partner:** Share your goals with a friend, family member, or support group member to hold you accountable. Regular check-ins can be motivating and encouraging.

3. **Listen to Your Body:** Monitor how different foods and activities impact your blood sugar levels. Keep a notebook to record your food, physical activity, and blood sugar levels. This might help you detect patterns and make informed decisions.

4. **Be Flexible:** Accept that setbacks may occur. Rather than being discouraged, see setbacks as chances to learn and improve. Adjust your plan as needed while remaining focused on your long-term goals.

5. **Practice Mindfulness:** Incorporate mindfulness practices into your everyday routine to reduce stress and improve general well-being. This can include meditation, deep breathing exercises, or simply taking a few minutes each day to reflect on your progress.

Success in blood sugar management is a journey full of ups and downs, but the community's experiences and insights can be invaluable. You can construct a long-term health plan by learning from others' inspiring testimonials, tackling common challenges, and implementing practical advice. Remember, you are not alone on this road; together, we can achieve long-term success.

Conclusion

Recap of Key Takeaways

As we conclude our investigation of the Blood Sugar Diet Solution, it's vital to consider the major lessons that can help you on your path to better health:

1. **Understanding Blood Sugar:** Proper blood sugar management is essential for sustaining good health. Understanding the role of insulin and the effects of different meals will help you make more informed dietary decisions.

2. **Identifying Issues:** Monitoring blood sugar levels and recognizing symptoms are crucial for early detection and action. Regular self-monitoring keeps you on track.

3. **Nutrition Fundamentals:** A well-balanced diet rich in macronutrients, vitamins, minerals, and fiber is crucial for managing blood sugar well. It is also important to consider meal timing and frequency.

4. **Meal Planning:** Creating a personalized blood sugar-friendly meal plan can help simplify decision-making and improve diet adherence. Portion control and understanding of dietary choices are essential for success.

5. **Positive Choices:** Consuming blood sugar-stabilizing foods and avoiding high-glycemic index and processed foods can significantly improve general health and well-being.

6. **Lifestyle Adjustments:** A holistic approach to blood sugar management includes physical activity, stress management, sleep prioritization, and support system building.

7. **Monitoring and Adaptation:** Regularly tracking progress and adapting to results is key to long-term success. Knowing when to seek professional help guarantees that you obtain the assistance you require.

8. **Community Support:** Connecting with people on similar journeys can boost motivation, offer tips, and create a sense of belonging. Learning from other people's experiences can be an effective strategy for conquering obstacles.

Encouragement for the Journey Ahead

Taking on the task of regulating blood sugar levels is both a struggle and an opportunity for growth. While you may have challenges along the way, realize that every minor change benefits your overall health. Celebrate your accomplishments, learn from your setbacks, and stay focused on your goals. Your commitment to improving your blood sugar management demonstrates your strength and resilience.

Remember, this journey is about more than just hitting particular numbers on a glucose monitor; it's about improving your quality of life. Adopting healthy behaviors is an investment in your future well-being and empowers you to live a full and active life.

Resources for Continued Support

To help you throughout your journey, here are some great resources for ongoing support:

1. **Books and Cookbooks:**
   - "The Diabetes Code" by Dr. Jason Fung
   - "Diabetes Meal Planning and Nutrition for Dummies" by American Diabetes Association
   - "The Blood Sugar Solution" by Dr. Mark Hyman
2. **Online Communities and Forums:**
   - Diabetes Daily: A supportive community offering resources and discussions.
   - The American Diabetes Association: A wealth of information on managing diabetes and local events.
   - Reddit's r/diabetes: An active forum for sharing experiences and advice.

3. **Mobile Apps:**
   - MySugr: A diabetes management app that helps track blood sugar levels, meals, and medications.
   - Carb Manager: A tool for tracking carbohydrate intake and meal planning.
   - Glucose Buddy: An app for logging blood sugar, medications, and meals.
4. **Professional Support:**
   - Consider connecting with a registered dietitian specializing in diabetes management for personalized meal planning and support.
   - Joining a local support group or diabetes education program can provide invaluable resources and encouragement.

As you continue on your journey, keep in mind that every step you take to manage your blood sugar is a step closer to a healthier, happier self. Stay informed, seek help, and celebrate the positive changes you're implementing for your health and well-being. You have got this!